Dreadful Beauty

Amy McKnight

Copyright © 2022 by Amy McKnight Unlimitted LLC

All rights reserved.

No portion of this book may be reproduced in any form without written permission from the publisher or author, except as permitted by U.S. copyright law.

Contents

Who Should Read This Book	1
My Promise to You	5
Introduction	6
1. Getting Started With Your Why	10
Questions to Consider Before Dreading	
Dealing with Family & Friends	
Reflections to Action	
2. Preparing Your Hair To Lock	14
Make Sure Your Hair is Long Enough	
Getting A Clean Start	
Pre-Installation Hair Prep	
Products To Avoid	

    Reflection to Action

3. Getting Your Sections Sorted   19
    Why The Size of Your Sections Matters
    Perfect Parts to Organic Sections
    Professional Parting Help is Worth It
    Why You Should Consider Getting a Friend to Help You
    How to See the Back Of Your Head
    Reflection to Action

4. Your Dreadlock Installation   31
    The Consultation
    The Lead-Up
    The Day/Night Before
    What to Bring & What Not to Bring
    Tools That Are Generally Used
    A Note on Separating/Parting
    Tangling
    Shaping
    Containing via Crocheting
    To Close or Not to Close (Your Tips)
    After Locking Care
    Reflection to Action

5. Maintenance: Taking care of your investment   48

    The Consultation
    The Lead-Up
    The Day/Night Before
    What to Bring and What Not to Bring
    Tools That are Generally Used
    A Note on Separating/Parting
    Tangling
    Shaping
    Containing via Crocheting
    To Close or Not to Close (Your Tips)
    After Locking Care
    Reflection to Action

6. Recipes for Healthy Dreads   65

    Conditioning with Natural Oils
    Herbs & Essential Oils
    Natural Hair Lightening & Coloring
    Acid Rinses
    Herbal Rinses & Refreshing Sprays
    Dreadlock Detox

7. Styling Your Lovely Locks   75

     Getting Started with Style
     Accent Locks & Wraps
     Adding Length At the Tips
     Adding Volume with Extensions
     The Beauty of Braid-In Extension
     Caring for Braid-in Extensions

8. When Things Go Wrong   84
     Dissatisfaction with Your Locks
     Thinning/Weak Dreads
     Mold in Your Dreads
     Super Skinny Dreads
     Loopy Bumpy Dreads
     Frizzy Locks
     Uneven Dreads
     Removing Dreadlocks

9. How We Help People Get Beautiful Dreads   91
     We Give Educated Guidance

10. The Next Step   95
     Don't Lose Your Momentum

Bibliography   99

Acknowledgments   103

Fullpage Image	108
About Amy McKnight	109
Also By Amy McKnight	111
About the Dreadful Beauty Podcast	112
A Small Request	113

Who Should Read This Book

This is an intentionally short book with all the fluff and filler removed, designed to be read in a single setting so you can gain insights as quickly as possible. Still, I don't want to waste your time if it is not a good fit. So, please take a few moments to read this entire section to see if the *Dreadful Beauty* book is an intelligent investment of your time, energy, and focus. I wrote this short book for the following reasons:

- To provide a concise and comprehensive guide on what it takes to start and maintain dreads on straight or wavy hair.

- To provide DIYers a framework of best practices to avoid the pitfalls.

- To invite you to consider connecting with a professional dreadlock artist like myself to determine if getting help with starting and/or maintaining your dreads is the best next step for you.

I've tried to distill and write out the best practices of dreadlocks and locking. If you are inclined, you can start and maintain your dreads yourself. However, most readers will be best served and have better dreadlocking outcomes if they reach out to a professional to see if getting help would make sense.

Three "types" of people are ideal readers for this book.

- This book is for people with straight or wavy hair looking to have dreadlocks installed and who want to know all they can before doing it.

- This book is for people who are at the beginning of their thought process towards getting dreads and are looking for a thorough overview of what the process will entail and pitfalls to avoid.

- This book is for people looking for a guide on maintaining their dreads on their own.

Finally, the *Dreadful Beauty* book was written for the person who agrees with these beliefs:

- Anyone who desires to wear dreads is free to do so regardless of race, creed, religion, or background.

- Although dreadlocks are essentially matted hair. It is purposefully matted hair. Neglect or uncleanness is not a necessary part of having dreads.

- Products can sometimes be helpful but are rarely absolutely necessary to achieve a beautiful set of dreads.

- Hair is hair. The vast principles that have allowed millions of people in ages past to present to lock their hair are still applicable today.

- It's ok to disagree. We all come to life with different backgrounds and experiences. We can still be friends.

Are we on the same page? Great! This book is for you. I sincerely appreciate you taking the time to continue this journey with me.

My Promise to You

When done correctly, dreadlocks look stunning on straight or wavy hair. I believe the information outlined in this book will help you start on the right foot if you are just starting out. If you have dreads and are not entirely satisfied with them, it can help you see where you may be going wrong.

By implementing the ideas in this book, you can take care of your dreads or have the tools to find someone to help you maintain them if you don't want to do it on your own.

Introduction

I get it. Finding clear, straightforward information on starting and maintaining dreads can be hard to get in one place.

I wanted a book like this for my hair texture in 2001 when I installed my first set of locks.

I didn't know it then, but it would be more than 20 years before I would find the method that works for my lifestyle, temperament, and hair. During that time, I would have many false starts and cumulative months of tediously removing sets that weren't quite right.

I have had a love-hate relationship with my hair for as long as I can remember. My hair is very thick and

GROWS when left to its own devices. Two things prized in the African American community.

However, like most black Americans, I have a mixed heritage that sometimes appears in our hair. The back and sides of my hair are perfectly coily and thick. However, the top is neither curly nor straight, has tiny rippled waves, and is less dense.

I would not be writing this book if my hair was all one texture, and I would probably be a very different person and would not have locks.

Nevertheless, my hair is mixed. In big and little ways, my fight to find a way to make the two diverse textures make peace has played a more significant part in my life than I'd like to admit.

Why am I sharing this? It has been a long road to get here, and on my 20+ year journey to having a peaceful existence with my hair through locks and locking, I've had to learn a lot. I've had some hair horror stories. I've been taken advantage of, misled, and misinformed.

So I have a profound empathy for anyone who feels like they are hitting wall after wall in their attempt at something quite simple - intentionally controlled tangled hair.

There is no product I would put in my hair that could make the rippled/wavy hair at the top of my hair lock on its own. That made me have to look for alternative natural solutions early on.

That biased me towards product-free locking methods for myself and others and ultimately brought me into the world of straight hair locking.

What follows is what I:

- Learned in the school of hard knocks,

- Observed over years of doing natural hair as a side hustle,

- Studied during my time in the Natural Hair Care Specialist school.

- Learned through much extracurricular training with various master loctician across the locking and dreading spectrum.

I think I bring a unique perspective to the topic. Hopefully, it can save you some of the hassle and heartache I've endured.

Chapter One

Getting Started With Your Why

If you are like most people, the decision to lock your hair isn't something you have come to quickly, and it is most likely a decision that has taken months to years to embrace.

So I'm not going to spend too much time telling you the importance of thinking about the emotional, financial, social, and other costs of starting dreads. I'm going to instead have you consider practical lifestyle questions.

Questions to Consider Before Dreading

Here are a few questions to think about as you are preparing to get dreads:

- Are you in the habit of going to the salon, or do you usually DIY? If you go to the salon, have you found a professional to help you along your dreading process?

- How often are you accustomed to shampooing your hair?

- Do you currently have any scalp conditions?

- Is your hair currently healthy? If not, is it damaged, dry, or brittle?

- Is your hair short, medium, or long? Are you prepared to see yourself with shorter hair? Are you ready to manage shorter hair? If not, have you factored in the cost of getting extensions?

- What is your lifestyle like? Are you an artist, an athlete, a student, a business professional, or self-employed?

- What hobbies and extracurricular activities are essential to you? Do you frequent the gym, swim, or work outdoors?

- What look are you ultimately going for? Do you want to make a statement? Or do you just want to simplify your life?

There are no "right" or "wrong" answers. But I would encourage you to grab a notebook and take a moment to write down your answers. As we continue on in the book, you may be more aware of how dreading your hair may impact your life based on the answers you give.

Dealing with Family & Friends

You probably already know this, but everyone has their own opinion of dreadlocks, locking, and lock wearers. So by extension, they will transfer those opinions to you. This is true even of friends and family who have known you all your life.

Depending on your personality, you may or may not care. But even for the most self-assured, it is hard to face criticism, questioning, and confrontation, especially when it comes from friends and family.

You can "just do it" and let the chips fall where they may. This is easier when you don't have to deal with people who disagree with your decision daily.

You might also consider trying to get some of your loved ones on board or at least gauge the future response by trying out temporary dreadlocks. It may be easier to deal with thoughtless comments when you haven't invested much time in natural dreads, which is a relatively permanent style.

When you go through with locking, you can use the temporary dreads to accentuate your natural dreads.

Reflections to Action

What is your "why"? If you haven't already written down the answers to the questions asked above. If your family isn't fully on board, think about how you can have a support system or network in place of dreadlock-friendly people to encourage you as you begin your locking journey.

Chapter Two

Preparing Your Hair To Lock

You've decided to get dreadlocks! Yay! Whether a dreadlock artist is installing them or you are DIYing, here are some principles and guidelines to keep in mind to ensure you have the best start.

Make Sure Your Hair is Long Enough

Most professional dreadlock artists can start dreads on hair that is at least 3-inches long. However, 5" to 6" is the generally preferred length. If your hair is:

- shorter overall

- growing out of a cut (especially mullet styles)

You may want to wait until your hair is at length before DIYing or scheduling your appointment. This will avoid the undesirable outcome of having very short locs at the top!

Getting A Clean Start

The next thing you want to do is ensure you get a clean start. This not only refers to cleansing the hair but also starting out with your hair in the best condition it can be. So it is a good idea to:

- Get a trim if you have split ends or damaged hair.

- Do any hair coloring now so as not to need to do it when your dreads are very new and fragile.

- Get rid of any products you will not use on your new dreads.

- Purchase dread-friendly shampoo to be used in the next step.

Pre-Installation Hair Prep

If you are accustomed to shampooing your hair daily, going one to 1 - 2 times a week will be a significant shock to your scalp. A gentler approach to cutting down on shampooing is to gradually work your way down to less frequent shampoo over a few weeks to a month.

How long you take depends on when you are scheduled to install your locks. The more time you can allow for adjusting to the change is better. Cutting down one wash a week over several months is ideal.

Here is a possible schedule if you are very short on time:

- Week 1 - Wash your hair every other day.

- Sunday/Tuesday/Thursday/Saturday

- Week 2 - Wash your hair every 2nd day

- Sunday/Wednesday/Saturday

- Week 3- Wash your hair every 2 - 3 days, Sunday and Thursday

You may experience excessive oiliness. This is normal. Your scalp is just trying to figure out what you are doing. Once you get into a routine, it will calm down. It is better to get it sorted now than when you have your new dreads.

When doing your shampooing, you want to use a dreadlock-friendly shampoo which is also healthier for you and your hair. That is a shampoo that is free of:

- Sodium lauryl sulfates/Sodium Laureth Sulfate (SLS/SLES) - Makes foam and bubbles.

- Parabens -Preservative. Linked to breast cancer

- Propylene glycol - Conditioner/softener. Linked to irritation and reactions.

- Phthalates - Softener. Linked to toxins.

Products To Avoid

In addition to avoiding shampoo with the ingredients above, you want to wean yourself off of using conditioners. This may seem scary. But the fantastic thing about shampoos that are good for locks is that they are better for your brushable hair.

Many of the ingredients cause stripping of the hair, and conditioners are needed to compensate.

Also, you'll want to start to wean yourself off using gels, balms, holding sprays, etc. This will give you the cleanest palate to have dreads created on.

Reflection to Action

What, if anything, do you need to do to prepare your hair for dreadlock installation?

Chapter Three

Getting Your Sections Sorted

Even if you are not doing your locks yourself, you may want to have a basic understanding of how you want your locks sectioned. This is especially true if you cannot work with a professional dreadlock artist and are working with someone to have dreads started for you.

Next to how your hair is initially tangled, the section size and layout will make a big difference in how your overall dreadlocks look.

Why The Size of Your Sections Matters

Section size deserves more than a little bit of thought for many reasons. Here are just a few:

- The weight of your future dreadlocks will be suspended on the sections of hair that are created at installation; you want it to be able to support it.

- The section size will ultimately determine the size and number of dreads.

- The number of locks will significantly impact the time you'll need to devote to maintenance.

- Sizing can be fixed to some extent in established locks, but it is best to get it as close to ideal as possible from the beginning.

So how big should you make the sections for your dreads? The density of your hair will help to determine that.

- The part sizing for average hair is about 1" x 1", which works out to about 60 - 70 dreads.

DREADFUL BEAUTY

- Thicker hair can accommodate smaller section sizes (less than 1" to .5") and more locks (80 to well over 100 dreads).

- Thinner hair should be parted slightly larger than an inch and will have fewer locks (usually less than 50)

Aside from density, you will want to think about your lifestyle.

- The more locks you have, the more maintenance you'll need to do or have done.

- Thin locks can quickly merge if you don't stay on top of separating them at their bases to keep them from joining together.

- Thin dreads often take longer to mature.

- Thick dreads tend to mature much quicker.

- Thicker locks can take a bit longer to dry. Something to consider if you swim or exercise a lot.

Those are just a few things that might make you choose one size over another.

Perfect Parts to Organic Sections

After you've decided on the size of your locks, you may want to think about how you want them arranged on your head. This is determined by the style or shape that they are parted in. The following are some common parting styles:

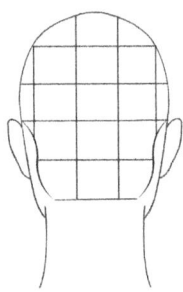

Grid - sections are arranged like grid paper. Very spacey - shows lots of your scalp. Works for thick hair and/or small dread sizes. Useful for styling that requires clean parting.

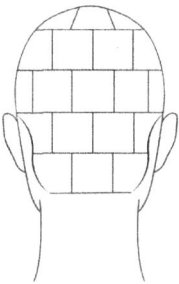

Bricklay- sections staggered so that the vertical lines are directly above the middle of the lock on the row below it. Good scalp coverage and works with any hair type.

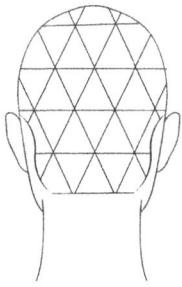

Triangle - Created by creating horizontal rows and dividing the sections with alternating diagonal partings. Good scalp coverage but is more tricky than brick.

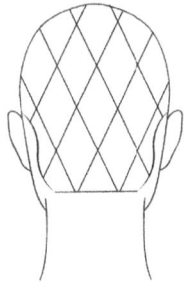

Diamond - Sections are created by making diagonal lines across the scalp. Dreads fall between dreads on the rows below. Most challenging pattern to execute.

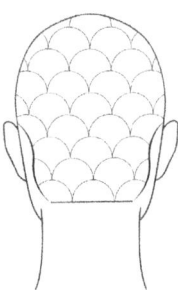

Fan/Half-moon/Crescent/Fish Scales - are similar to bricklaying in that the bottom of the subsequent locks are in the middle of the locks below it. Excellent scalp coverage and gives a structured organic look.

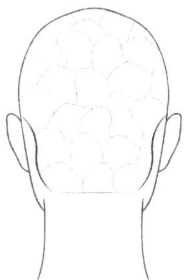

Grab and Go/Organic - Sections are grabbed with less effort to make the locks a particular shape while keeping sizing relatively the same.

The parting will depend on what you feel comfortable executing or what your artist offers.

Professional Parting Help is Worth It

The preceding information is a lot to take into consideration. And I know the feeling (and the relief) that comes from letting someone else figure it out and happily sitting in the salon chair.

Parting is so crucial to the locking process and the foundation of your locks that it is something that you want to have done by someone who can do it so that you don't second guess later on.

Suppose you cannot get to a professional dreadlock artist and plan to DIY. You might consider getting a local braider to part your hair in that case. Find a braider, not a loctician. There is no need to pay a premium for this.

Just ask for 60 large or 25 jumbo braids with extensions. Yes, you will take them out, but you will get better service and results if you let them create a style that will look nice when they are done. They can take a picture of you for their portfolio.

You don't need to explain why you want them and what you plan to do. In fact, it is probably best not to talk about it. Seriously. Not helpful. Why? Because you'll either confuse them or possibly bias them against you. Neither option will get you great results.

Check portfolios before calling around. You want someone who creates neat, consistent sections/parts. You will probably get bricklaying parts. If you want some other style, make sure it is something that they do regularly by looking at their portfolio.

They will want to use gel/ product on your hair. Bring a salon spray bottle with water, and tell them a natural hair care specialist you know (that would be me) told you that it was possible to part your hair with water instead of gel. Thank them for being willing to work with you.

In the next chapter, we will discuss how to create the actual locks in depth, so I'll not cover that here. What you will do is take down each individual braid and backcomb or twist and rip the section and proceed from there. Being in braids will actually give you a little extra texture to your hair and could aid in backcombing.

Why You Should Consider Getting a Friend to Help You

No local braiders? No problem. Ask a friend to help you. Seriously, going it alone is so not fun.

If you are a DIYer, this is the part, even more so than locking, where you might want to think about getting help. In theory, you just draw lines across your scalp with a comb. In practice, you want those lines and sections to be even and relatively consistent. That is way more challenging than you might suspect.

I have had to part my hair for various styles, including installing my own sets of locks. On every occasion, somewhere along the line, I would think. I wish I had someone to help me. EVERY. SINGLE. TIME.

The second pair of eyes and hands can give you peace of mind, and it will also cut the process in half as you are not having to consult mirrors and contort your body to get your parts right.

The simplest thing is to let them section and rubber band your whole head. If anything needs to be tweaked later, you can do that after they've done the most challenging part for you.

How to See the Back Of Your Head

No pro, friend, or family to help you? I hear you. I've been there. This is the method I used to install 350 micro-sized locks with precise grid sectioning on myself. It was a grind. But it worked so well that people thought they were done by someone else.

It really wasn't a complicated setup. Here's what you will need:

DREADFUL BEAUTY

- Your phone

- Screen mirroring app for your phone

- Way to position the phone behind your head. (Arkon mount, selfie stick, etc.)

- A computer or tablet

- Wifi

You'll download the app on your phone and open it. It will give you an address to put into a browser's address bar. Put that into the tablet or computer, which should be facing you.

Click "Start Mirroring" on your phone. Refresh the page on your computer and/or tablet. You should see whatever is on your phone screen. Navigate to your camera and open the photo like you were going to take a picture. Now position the phone so that it is behind your head, pointing to the area you need to see.

Walah! You have eyes on the back of your head.

You're welcome!

Reflection to Action

What size and parting shape are you leaning towards for your dreadlocks?

Chapter Four

Your Dreadlock Installation

Getting your dreads installed is such a super exciting time! In this chapter, we will be looking at what you can expect if you are going to get it professionally done. We will also look at the basic installation process if you want to do it yourself.

The Consultation

If you have your locks done by a professional dreadlock artist, you will probably have filled out an online form. That lets them understand a little about you, your hair history, what you are looking for in your new installation, and whether you want extensions, decorations, etc.

During your initial new client consultation, the two of you will review your answers to ensure everyone is on the same page.

This is an excellent opportunity for you to get any questions you may have about the process answered. It is also the opportunity for both of you to interview each other. Yes, there is a high possibility that they may be interviewing you. To make sure that you are a good fit. You will spend several hours together in a close setting and must be comfortable.

It is more than likely you will be fine. The locked community tends to attract people with a similar vibe.

There may be a fee for the consultation. Sometimes that will go towards the cost of your installation. Sometimes it is a separate service.

When everything is done, you will probably be asked to put down a portion of the estimated cost of installation to book the date. If you are ordering extensions, you will generally be asked to pay for those up front if they are custom-made.

Once those things are taken care of, and the date is on the calendar, you're set!

You will want to be aware of the cancelation policy. Things happen, and canceling might be unavoidable. You will want to know how much notice is needed to cancel/change the date and how funds already paid will be handled.

The Lead-Up

During the consultation, they will likely tell you how they would have you prepare for the installation and what products they recommend. You'll want to take notes of these instructions and follow them to have the best installation experience.

The Day/Night Before

Whether flying in from out of town or driving up the road, it is a good idea to have as restful a day as possible and a good night's sleep the night before. Though it might be hard to sleep for excitement!

It isn't a bad idea to start drinking water if you are not in the habit of doing that. Dehydration can intensify the feeling of pain. Your scalp and body will thank you.

What to Bring & What Not to Bring

As you think about what to pack, remember you'll be sitting for long periods. So bring something so that you'll be comfortable.

- Ensure your digital devices are charged, and you have the cords and blocks you need. They may have water and snacks, but bringing some of your own isn't a bad idea, especially if you have special dietary needs.

- They may stop to let you both take lunch or work straight through and have you eat in the chair. If the salon isn't close to places that deliver, it might be a good idea to pack lunch. This is an excellent question to ask during the consultation.

- Projects and hobbies that can be done on your lap if that is your type of thing can also be good.

- If you have low pain tolerance, you may consider taking some medication for pain before the service starts and at the proper interval during and after.

- Of course, bring a positive, happy attitude!

What not to bring is as important as what to bring, or at least ask before showing up with:

- Children - Except for a baby that will be content being held on your lap, bringing kids isn't a good idea.

- Extra people - unless it is explicitly stated on their website that you are welcome to bring a friend, don't assume it is ok.

- Pets aren't allowed in a salon environment in most states, and people may not want them in their homes.

- A bad attitude.

You want your artist to do fun, creative work. You need to feed that with good energy.

Tools That Are Generally Used

Each dreadlock artist will have their own method of installing dreadlocks depending on the processes used to tangle, shape, and then contain the tangled hair.

- Tangling - usually done either by backcombing or twisting and pulling/ripping or a combination of both.

  - Tools needed: one of the following - fine tooth comb, rat-tailed comb/ flea comb/ metal dread comb.

- Shaped - done by palm rolling

  - hands

- Contained - Pre-locking - done by crocheting and/or micro-latch hooking

Tools needed one or more of the following:

- 1.00/0.75/0.6/0.5/0.45 mm steel crochet hook (Clover is my preferred brand). You may also see/use a micro-latch hook

* (Optional) Rubber Bands/Elastic bands for sectioning - removed during/after installation.

Some may do each part of the process over the entire head before proceeding to the next part. While others may do one dread at a time. There is no right or wrong way, and each artist will have their own preference.

A Note on Separating/Parting

I covered how to section your dreads in the previous chapter to keep this chapter from being so overwhelming. However, before the following steps were done, the decision of how the hair section would be section would have been made.

Some dreadlock artists will section the entire head before proceeding to the next steps. Others will section as they go, and some may do both.

If you are doing your hair yourself, it is not a bad idea to have your hair sectioned before you start and then go back and do the work.

In natural hair care school, when we needed a precise number of braids in some situations, we would section a client's hair before starting.

I tell you this because most, if not all, of us had years, and some of us had decades of doing hair under our belts before attending school. We went to get the paper that allowed us to have the ability to formally work in salons.

I share this because there is no shame in sectioning beforehand. We did that for styles usually taken out in a few weeks. Why not take the time to plan for a style that you may be wearing for years?

Tangling

Once your hair has been sectioned, it is time for it to be tangled. This can be done in one or a combination of two main ways. Backcombing and/ or twist and pull (aka twist and rip)

Backcombing

In backcombing, hair is teased from the root to the scalp to create tangles, and this is the basis of creating dreads in straight hair.

This is a critical step. Improper backcombing at the beginning can lead to areas of thin, weak, and or uneven dreads and or dreads with loops, angles, elbows, and bumps as the hair dreads unevenly.

If you are DIYing your locks, you'll want to take care to evenly tease the hair. You don't want to have areas where there are long portions of undreaded hair. This can happen when you are not teasing evenly all around, and one side is more teased than the other.

If you are DIYing, you might want to get some Kanekalon synthetic bulk hair. It can be purchased at ethnic beauty supply stores, online, and/or human extension hair on the weft.

Attach it to something stationary, and then practice backcombing the hair evenly until you get your technique down. You'll probably want to do it before the day you are doing your installation. If you have a friend that will be helping you with this part, see if you can get them to practice with you.

Backcombing seems the most common way of tangling straight or wavy hair to start dreads. So much so that among traditional/ afro-hair loctician, dreads created on straight hair are often referred to as "backcombed dreads." However, it is not the only way to make the tangles that will be the foundation for your dreads.

If you don't see a tool for backcombing on your dreadlock artist table, it isn't because they are out of the loop. They may use a different but effective method to create tangles. They may twist and pull.

Twist & Pull (AKA Twist & Rip)

The twist and pull method is another means of creating tangles that turn into locks. The hair is twisted, then separated so that knots are created and driven towards the base of your hair, and it is done until you have tangles down the length of the hair.

Some dreadlock artists love this method, and others have sworn off it. Each artist has their own reasons.

It seems that dreads created with the twist and pull method are sometimes a little slimmer than dreads of the same section size that have been backcombed. But crocheting methods will play a part in how compact the final dread will be.

Twist and Pull seems to be popular among DIYers. It makes sense as it is easier to do on yourself than backcombing, especially for hard-to-reach areas of your head.

Again, if you plan to DIY, getting some synthetic or human hair to practice the technique before attempting it on your own head will not hurt.

Shaping

After the hair has been tangled by some means, you will have a bit of a fuzzy mess. The fuzziness will depend on the method used and proficiency with the technique.

It is at this point some, but not all, dreadlock artists may palm roll your hair into a more cylindrical form before containing it all with crocheting.

Containing via Crocheting

A long time ago, before we all knew better, this was the point where wax would be applied to "hold the hair together." Gratefully we are all older and wiser and realize there is a much more effective way of containing the hair and encouraging the dread to hold its shape. This method has none of the many cons of wax and holding products.

There are many ways to crochet your hair. Your dreadlock artist will have the method that they use. The one in the adjacent state (or country) may do something different. The goal is to keep the hair together so the dreads can be washed without disintegrating and coming untangled.

In the course of my personal education in this area, I've learned several ways to effectively crochet straight hair. There are similarities and differences between them all. They seem to fall into 3 main groups:

- Some methods **draw the loose hair into the body** of the forming dreadlock.

Other methods **wrap the hair around the body** of the forming dreadlock.

- Still, other techniques are a **mixture of both.**

I'm not going more in-depth than this. Some of what I learned in this area is proprietary to the creators of the method.

If you are a DIYer, just that categorization should remove some of the confusion you may have when watching youtube videos of people crocheting. Some will spell out what they are doing, and others expect you to get it. Everyone isn't doing the same thing. But most are doing a version of the above.

Crocheting, like backcombing, twisting, and pulling, is usually done from root to tip. As you or your dreadlock artist gets to the ends of your lock, you'll have one last decision to make:

To Close or Not to Close (Your Tips)

If you have extensions attached to the ends of your locks for length. The tips will be left open to connect extension locks or create dreads as needed on the spot, depending on your situation.

If your hair is long or you don't need/want extensions added, you'll have to decide how you want your tips.

There are pros and cons to both options.

- Closing your tips can be an extra safeguard against your hair trying to come undreaded. This is especially true if you have very straight hair that is highly resistant to locking. However, it can shorten your locks by 1-3 inches.

- Leaving your tips open will give you more length and "soften" the looks of dreads. But you will need to take time to care for the ends so that they don't inadvertently become matted in a way you don't want.

- Closed tips dry a little slower than open tips, but not enough to make a huge difference.

In the end, it will probably come down to aesthetics which way you think you'll be most comfortable. And you may not be able to make that decision until you look at your new dreads.

After Locking Care

Your locks are in! Now what? Your dreadlock artist will have their own aftercare instructions for you. Which may include their recommended products which they may carry.

Your hair and scalp may feel uncomfortable or painful. This is especially true if this is the first time you've had this type of service done to your hair. If you have had braid-in-locks or some other braid/extension service done before, you may be a little more prepared for the potential discomfort.

Those painkillers that you may have taken may be wearing off. If you know you don't do well with pain or suffer from tension headaches, you may want to take something before getting on the road.

Over the next few days, expect your scalp and hair to change as it settles into this new state.

You may also need to "settle into" your new look. The euphoria that is present at your installation may wane. Especially if you get grief from family and friends about your decision.

You'll want to take care of your own mental health. You may want to seek some support before your installation. A support system will be able to encourage you on days when your locks aren't doing or looking quite like you hope.

It is not uncommon to experience a bit of "buyer's remorse" a few days or even weeks after getting your installation. Did you make the right decisions? Should your locks be smaller (or bigger)? Is too much scalp showing? All the things.

It's ok.

It can happen when you make a choice that isn't easily undone and will pass. Remember your why, and have some pretty scarves and head wraps on hand! It is amazing how a scarf around the hairline can change the look!

You made a good decision, and you didn't make it lightly. You'll look back and wonder why you didn't do it sooner. I promise.

Reflection to Action

After reading this chapter, what questions might you want to discuss with a dreadlock artist before your installation? How do you feel about the process? As you picture yourself going through the process, what would you need to do to ensure you have the best experience possible?

Chapter Five

Maintenance: Taking Care of Your Investment

Getting your dreads installed is such a super exciting time! In this chapter, we will be looking at what you can expect if you are going to get it professionally done. We will also look at the basic installation process if you want to do it yourself.

The Consultation

If you have your locks done by a professional dreadlock artist, you will probably have filled out an online form.

That lets them understand a little about you, your hair history, what you are looking for in your new installation, and whether you want extensions, decorations, etc.

During your initial new client consultation, the two of you will review your answers to ensure everyone is on the same page.

This is an excellent opportunity for you to get any questions you may have about the process answered. It is also the opportunity for both of you to interview each other. Yes, there is a high possibility that they may be interviewing you. To make sure that you are a good fit. You will spend several hours together in a close setting and must be comfortable.

It is more than likely you will be fine. The locked community tends to attract people with a similar vibe.

There may be a fee for the consultation. Sometimes that will go towards the cost of your installation. Sometimes it is a separate service.

When everything is done, you will probably be asked to put down a portion of the estimated cost of installation to book the date. If you are ordering extensions, you will generally be asked to pay for those up front if they are custom-made.

Once those things are taken care of, and the date is on the calendar, you're set!

You will want to be aware of the cancelation policy. Things happen, and canceling might be unavoidable. You will want to know how much notice is needed to cancel/change the date and how funds already paid will be handled.

The Lead-Up

During the consultation, they will likely tell you how they would have you prepare for the installation and what products they recommend. You'll want to take notes of these instructions and follow them to have the best installation experience.

The Day/Night Before

Whether flying in from out of town or driving up the road, it is a good idea to have as restful a day as possible and a good night's sleep the night before. Though it might be hard to sleep for excitement!

It isn't a bad idea to start drinking water if you are not in the habit of doing that. Dehydration can intensify the feeling of pain. Your scalp and body will thank you.

What to Bring and What Not to Bring

As you think about what to pack, remember you'll be sitting for long periods. So bring something so that you'll be comfortable.

- Ensure your digital devices are charged, and you have the cords and blocks you need. They may have water and snacks, but bringing some of your own isn't a bad idea, especially if you have special dietary needs.

- They may stop to let you both take lunch or work straight through and have you eat in the chair. If the salon isn't close to places that deliver, it might be a good idea to pack lunch. This is an excellent question to ask during the consultation.

- Projects and hobbies that can be done on your lap if that is your type of thing can also be good.

- If you have low pain tolerance, you may consider taking some medication for pain before the service starts and at the proper interval during and after.

- Of course, bring a positive, happy attitude!

What not to bring is as important as what to bring, or at least ask before showing up with:

- Children - Except for a baby that will be content being held on your lap, bringing kids isn't a good idea.

- Extra people - unless it is explicitly stated on their website that you are welcome to bring a friend, don't assume it is ok.

- Pets aren't allowed in a salon environment in most states, and people may not want them in their homes.

- A bad attitude.

You want your artist to do fun, creative work. You need to feed that with good energy.

Tools That are Generally Used

Each dreadlock artist will have their own method of installing dreadlocks depending on the processes used to tangle, shape, and then contain the tangled hair.

- Tangling - usually done either by backcombing or twisting and pulling/ripping or a combination of both.

  - Tools needed: one of the following - fine tooth comb, rat-tailed comb/ flea comb/ metal dread comb.

- Shaped - done by palm rolling

  - hands

- Contained - Pre-locking - done by crocheting and/or micro-latch hooking

Tools needed one or more of the following:

- 1.00/0.75/0.6/0.5/0.45 mm steel crochet hook (Clover is my preferred brand). You may also see/use a micro-latch hook

- (Optional) Rubber Bands/Elastic bands for sectioning - removed during/after installation.

Some may do each part of the process over the entire head before proceeding to the next part. While others may do one dread at a time. There is no right or wrong way, and each artist will have their own preference.

A Note on Separating/Parting

I covered how to section your dreads in the previous chapter to keep this chapter from being so overwhelming. However, before the following steps were done, the decision of how the hair section would be section would have been made.

Some dreadlock artists will section the entire head before proceeding to the next steps. Others will section as they go, and some may do both.

If you are doing your hair yourself, it is not a bad idea to have your hair sectioned before you start and then go back and do the work.

In natural hair care school, when we needed a precise number of braids in some situations, we would section a client's hair before starting.

I tell you this because most, if not all, of us had years, and some of us had decades of doing hair under our belts before attending school. We went to get the paper that allowed us to have the ability to formally work in salons.

I share this because there is no shame in sectioning beforehand. We did that for styles usually taken out in a few weeks. Why not take the time to plan for a style that you may be wearing for years?

Tangling

Once your hair has been sectioned, it is time for it to be tangled. This can be done in one or a combination of two main ways. Backcombing and/ or twist and pull (aka twist and rip)

Backcombing

In backcombing, hair is teased from the root to the scalp to create tangles, and this is the basis of creating dreads in straight hair.

This is a critical step. Improper backcombing at the beginning can lead to areas of thin, weak, and or uneven dreads and or dreads with loops, angles, elbows, and bumps as the hair dreads unevenly.

If you are DIYing your locks, you'll want to take care to evenly tease the hair. You don't want to have areas where there are long portions of undreaded hair. This can happen when you are not teasing evenly all around, and one side is more teased than the other.

If you are DIYing, you might want to get some Kanekalon synthetic bulk hair. It can be purchased at ethnic beauty supply stores, online, and/or human extension hair on the weft.

Attach it to something stationary, and then practice backcombing the hair evenly until you get your technique down. You'll probably want to do it before the day you are doing your installation. If you have a friend that will be helping you with this part, see if you can get them to practice with you.

Backcombing seems the most common way of tangling straight or wavy hair to start dreads. So much so that among traditional/ afro-hair loctician, dreads created on straight hair are often referred to as "backcombed dreads." However, it is not the only way to make the tangles that will be the foundation for your dreads.

If you don't see a tool for backcombing on your dreadlock artist table, it isn't because they are out of the loop. They may use a different but effective method to create tangles. They may twist and pull.

Twist & Pull (AKA Twist & Rip)

The twist and pull method is another means of creating tangles that turn into locks. The hair is twisted, then separated so that knots are created and driven towards the base of your hair, and it is done until you have tangles down the length of the hair.

Some dreadlock artists love this method, and others have sworn off it. Each artist has their own reasons.

It seems that dreads created with the twist and pull method are sometimes a little slimmer than dreads of the same section size that have been backcombed. But crocheting methods will play a part in how compact the final dread will be.

Twist and Pull seems to be popular among DIYers. It makes sense as it is easier to do on yourself than backcombing, especially for hard-to-reach areas of your head.

Again, if you plan to DIY, getting some synthetic or human hair to practice the technique before attempting it on your own head will not hurt.

Shaping

After the hair has been tangled by some means, you will have a bit of a fuzzy mess. The fuzziness will depend on the method used and proficiency with the technique.

It is at this point some, but not all, dreadlock artists may palm roll your hair into a more cylindrical form before containing it all with crocheting.

Containing via Crocheting

A long time ago, before we all knew better, this was the point where wax would be applied to "hold the hair together." Gratefully we are all older and wiser and realize there is a much more effective way of containing the hair and encouraging the dread to hold its shape. This method has none of the many cons of wax and holding products.

There are many ways to crochet your hair. Your dreadlock artist will have the method that they use. The one in the adjacent state (or country) may do something different. The goal is to keep the hair together so the dreads can be washed without disintegrating and coming untangled.

In the course of my personal education in this area, I've learned several ways to effectively crochet straight hair. There are similarities and differences between them all. They seem to fall into 3 main groups:

- Some methods **draw the loose hair into the body** of the forming dreadlock.

Other methods **wrap the hair around the body** of the forming dreadlock.

- Still, other techniques are a **mixture of both.**

I'm not going more in-depth than this. Some of what I learned in this area is proprietary to the creators of the method.

If you are a DIYer, just that categorization should remove some of the confusion you may have when watching youtube videos of people crocheting. Some will spell out what they are doing, and others expect you to get it. Everyone isn't doing the same thing. But most are doing a version of the above.

Crocheting, like backcombing, twisting, and pulling, is usually done from root to tip. As you or your dreadlock artist gets to the ends of your lock, you'll have one last decision to make:

To Close or Not to Close (Your Tips)

If you have extensions attached to the ends of your locks for length. The tips will be left open to connect extension locks or create dreads as needed on the spot, depending on your situation.

If your hair is long or you don't need/want extensions added, you'll have to decide how you want your tips.

There are pros and cons to both options.

- Closing your tips can be an extra safeguard against your hair trying to come undreaded. This is especially true if you have very straight hair that is highly resistant to locking. However, it can shorten your locks by 1-3 inches.

- Leaving your tips open will give you more length and "soften" the looks of dreads. But you will need to take time to care for the ends so that they don't inadvertently become matted in a way you don't want.

- Closed tips dry a little slower than open tips, but not enough to make a huge difference.

In the end, it will probably come down to aesthetics which way you think you'll be most comfortable. And you may not be able to make that decision until you look at your new dreads.

After Locking Care

Your locks are in! Now what? Your dreadlock artist will have their own aftercare instructions for you. Which may include their recommended products which they may carry.

Your hair and scalp may feel uncomfortable or painful. This is especially true if this is the first time you've had this type of service done to your hair. If you have had braid-in-locks or some other braid/extension service done before, you may be a little more prepared for the potential discomfort.

Those painkillers that you may have taken may be wearing off. If you know you don't do well with pain or suffer from tension headaches, you may want to take something before getting on the road.

Over the next few days, expect your scalp and hair to change as it settles into this new state.

DREADFUL BEAUTY

You may also need to "settle into" your new look. The euphoria that is present at your installation may wane. Especially if you get grief from family and friends about your decision.

You'll want to take care of your own mental health. You may want to seek some support before your installation. A support system will be able to encourage you on days when your locks aren't doing or looking quite like you hope.

It is not uncommon to experience a bit of "buyer's remorse" a few days or even weeks after getting your installation. Did you make the right decisions? Should your locks be smaller (or bigger)? Is too much scalp showing? All the things.

It's ok.

It can happen when you make a choice that isn't easily undone and will pass. Remember your why, and have some pretty scarves and head wraps on hand! It is amazing how a scarf around the hairline can change the look!

You made a good decision, and you didn't make it lightly. You'll look back and wonder why you didn't do it sooner. I promise.

Reflection to Action

After reading this chapter, what questions might you want to discuss with a dreadlock artist before your installation? How do you feel about the process? As you picture yourself going through the process, what would you need to do to ensure you have the best experience possible?

Chapter Six

Recipes for Healthy Dreads

Herb and oils provide an excellent alternative to the usage of commercially made products. Many companies that cater to dreadheads create products from all-natural sources.

Are you into or interested in using common herbs, essential oils, vegetable oils, and natural botanicals? This chapter will give you additional resources you can use with your dreads.

Although many herbs and oils can be ingested, this chapter only covers their external application. Before applying any natural product, you should consider doing a patch test. And, of course, avoid anything to which you may be allergic.

Conditioning with Natural Oils

Although conditioners, as a rule, are a no-no when it comes to dreadlocks for a host of reasons. You may find that your dreads feel dry and brittle. This is because the natural oils from your scalp cannot travel down the length of your hair as they would if your hair were not in dreads but in a brushable state.

The solution is to use light natural oils as needed to supply the absence of the oils created by your scalp. When looking for an oil to use, you want to find something fast absorbing and liquid at room temperature.

No more than a thimble is needed for your entire head. Oil is best applied after shampooing while the hair is damp but not wet.

Some carrier oils that fit the bill are:

- **Apricot Seed Oil** - Softens dry hair

- **Avocado Oil** - Stimulates growth & restores dehydrated/damaged hair.

- **Fractionated Coconut Oil** - Regenerative, helps brittle hair.

- **Grapeseed Oil** - Moisturizes dry, brittle hair. Strengthens hair cuticle.

- **Sweet Almond Oil** - Reduces itching and inflammation.

Herbs & Essential Oils

Herbs and essential oils can also be a helpful addition to your maintenance schedule. Essential oils are best added to recipes at a 5% - 10% ratio because of their inherent natural potency.

Many beneficial herbs are used in herbal rinses and as hair oils. Here are a few commonly used with dreads and their benefits.

- **Peppermint** - Oily scalp, Anti-Dandruff, Astringent

- **Lavender** - Hair growth, cell rejuvenation, softener, conditioner, astringent

- **Rosemary** - Oily scalp, hair loss, hair growth, anti-dandruff, softener, conditioner, astringent

- **Tea tree** - Antiseptic, anti-dandruff, astringent

- **Lemon (juice)** - antiseptic, astringent

- **Eucalyptus** - Oily scalp, antiseptic, scalp soother, anti-dandruff,

- **Sage** - Antiseptic, hair loss, hair growth, scalp soothers, anti-dandruff, conditioner, astringent.

- **Basil** - Oily scalp, moisturizer, hair growth

- **Thyme** - Oily scalp, antiseptic, hair loss, hair growth, conditioner.

- **Chamomile** - Antiseptic, moisturizer, scalp soother, astringent

Natural Hair Lightening & Coloring

Herbs and the juices of fruits and plants have been used for millennia for dying. If you want a gradual change, the following recipes with a little time and sun can provide that.

Dark Coffee Hair Dye - Brew 2 - 3 cups of dark roast coffee double strength. Let cool. Using a bowl or basin to catch the liquid, saturate dreads until completely covered. Cover with a plastic bag and let sit for 1 hour. Rinse with cool water.

Lemon Juice Chamomile Hair Lightener - Add the juice of 1 lemon and a cup of double-brewed chamomile tea to a spray bottle. Spray on your hair and go out in the sun for 30 minutes. Lightning effects will depend on your hair's natural color.

Acid Rinses

Our hair/scalp's natural pH ranges from 4.5 to 5.5 on the pH scale, which is slightly acidic. Distilled water is 7, which is neutral, and ammonia is around 12.

Acid rinses can help to restore the hair's natural pH balance. They are also helpful in removing residual soap and debris from dreads.

If you want to make an acid rinse, any of the following ingredients can be mixed with water at a ratio of 95:5. Which is 95% water to 5% acid.

- Citric acids - lemon juice, lime juice, orange juice, grapefruit juice, cactus juice.

- Apple Cider Vinegar or Distilled Vinegar

- Tartaric acid - wine, champagne, beer (leave odors must be rinsed out)

Herbal Rinses & Refreshing Sprays

Herbal rinses are a natural residue-free way to condition and nourish your dreads. They can help address issues you may have with your scalp or dreads. Or they can be used cosmetically to enhance color or add fragrance.

The primary method for creating and using a herbal infusion for a rinse or spray is as follows:

- Mix herbs to be used in a bowl or french press

- Boil water and pour over herbs

- Let steep for 20 - 30 minutes or longer.

- Strain and add in cool water as needed if still hot.

- Pour into a bottle and add in any essential oils and shake.

The mixture can be used as the final rinse after shampooing, or it can be poured into a spray bottle, lightly sprayed on the scalp, and locks daily. Store in the fridge for up to a week.

Dreadlock Detox

A dread detox is a way of deep cleaning your locks to remove residue and debris that may not come out with regular washing.

It is very stripping to the hair as baking soda, which is alkaline, is used to help with the cleaning process. So it is not something you want to do more than once a quarter or at the change of the seasons.

If you are careful in what you put on your hair and avoid situations that would cause build-up, you may not need to have a dread detox done at all.

However, if you live in an area with hard water and have developed build-up, or your dreads smell moldy, dank, mildewy, or you've been swimming in freshwater ponds, lakes, or rivers, a dread detox may be necessary.

You will need the following to do a dread detox:

- A shampoo basin/large bowl/large new cat litter box big enough to contain your dreads and water to cover your dreads
- 6 ounces of apple cider vinegar
- Baking soda
- Empty gallon jug
- Towels
- Plastic sheeting (optional)

- A friend

Here is what you'll need to do:

- Protect areas with plastic sheeting if needed

- Fill basin/large bowl/large new, unused cat litter box with warm water

- Completely dissolve ½ cup of baking soda in the water.

- Pour ACV into the bottom of the empty gallon jug. Add water to fill. Set aside till final rinse.

- Lay with your dreads in the bowl.

- Have a friend pour baking soda water over your dreads and gently massage to ensure the mixture gets through.

- Remain with dreads submerged for 15 - 20 minutes.

You may see the water change colors. This is normal if you have residue and build-up in your dreads.

- At the end of the time, remove dreads from the liquid.

- Empty and rinse the basin.

- Rinse dreads well with clean water until it runs clear

- Do the final rinse with the ACV to neutralize residual baking soda in the shower or over the basin.

If you would rather get professional help than do this yourself, some dreadlock artists offer this and shampooing services.

Chapter Seven

Styling Your Lovely Locks

The sky's the limit to the styles you can do with your locks in and of themselves. When you start adding accents, temporary or permanent extensions, it goes out into the stratosphere.

Getting Started with Style

You can start styling and accessorizing your dreads from day one. Many dreadlock artists offer dreadlock decoration as a part of the installation/maintenance process, and some offer it as a separate service. During decoration, they may:

- Wrap your locks with yarn, fabric, ribbons, or twine.

- Add beads, charms, accent rings, or temporary synthetic/wool/human hair extensions (more on that below)

All in the service of taking your look up to the next level. These are also things that you can do yourself in between maintenance.

You'll probably want to get or have on-hand dreadlock-friendly hair ties, hats, and scrunchies for those times when you may want to pull your hair up or back. What makes an accessory dreadlock friendly? Here are a few characteristics:

- Large enough to accommodate hair without squeezing. - most accessories come in mm sizes. Measure your locks and find the size closest to your dread's diameter.

Made of material that doesn't snag or unnecessarily pull hair.

- Strong enough to hold locks without breaking

Accent Locks & Wraps

A simple way to add color and texture to natural dreadlocks is to accent them with criss-cross string wraps or add in premade decorated accent locks and wraps.

Accenting locks with yarn or floss is as simple as pulling off a length of a color or two. Doubling it and using the two legs plus the lock to make a three-strand braid. Wrap and tie when you come to the end of the yarn or dread.

When your locks are new, it is best to only use this wrap style as wraps that encase the whole dread without spaces create a hard-to-dry atmosphere, putting you at risk of mold and mildew in that wrapped lock.

A way to avoid this and still have a fully wrapped accented dread is to purchase or create accent dreadlock and festival wraps.

Simple accent dreadlocks can be made by braiding extension hair or yarn to a hair tie. Then decorate the faux lock with fabric, thread, floss, accents, etc. When you are done, it can be looped onto the base of a lock.

Friendship bracelet/macrame style wraps can also be attached to a hair tie and created

Adding Length At the Tips

Dreadlock extensions are a way to add seamless length to your hair and truly take your locks to the next level. All locks are cute. But there is something show-stopping about long dreadlocks.

Dreadlock extensions can be installed at the time of installation or later down the road if you want more length.

They are generally created beforehand for the sake of time. This is especially true for long lock extensions. However, some dreadlock artists will make dreads on the spot during installation time.

Like temporary extensions, they come in more than one type.

- Human hair - hair that is donated, collected, or purchased from human donors.

- Synthetic Hair - Kanekalon hair, as mentioned above.

Both human hair extension and synthetic extensions can be attached to the ends to give extra length, but there are pros and cons to each:

- Human hair - will most closely behave like your natural hair. It can be dyed (with care) and cared for like your natural dreads. It feels like hair - because it is hair. But lousy quality hair can create dreads that will not stand the test of time. Good quality hair is costly. Expect to pay as much, if not more, for your extensions as you pay for the installation. There is also the issue of unethical practices around collecting some hair types.

- Synthetic hair is inexpensive. And it is easy to find a variety of sets. It comes in a wide range of colors that do not fade. This can be a bad thing when your hair fades, and the extensions are the exact same color as day one. Bizarre look. Also, unfortunately, they can feel much less natural, and some people have an issue with the fact that they are made from petrochemicals.

Both human hair and synthetic extensions are usually installed on the ends of your natural dreads. This is done by using the crochet method overlapping your hair with the frayed end of the extensions. There is no need to glue, braid or use thread to hold it in.

When done by a skilled professional crochet specialist, the join is seamless with no lumps, bumps, or apparent connections. And it holds. You don't have to worry about walking down the street and losing a dread, and they are tight.

Adding Volume with Extensions

If you need a little more volume or extra flare, temporary extensions can do that for you. There are two main types of temporary extensions:

Synthetic - Usually made from Kanekalon braiding hair

- Wool - Made from the hair of sheep.

These usually come in two types which are:

- Double Ended (DE) - These extensions are twice as long as the intended length. So you are getting two instead of one. These are especially good for adding volume.

- A single End (SE) is a single extension with a loop at one end. These are good for adding accents without the added volume.

Temporary extensions come in a variety of colors, textures, and designs. There is a booming cottage industry of dreadlock extension artists, each with their own style and techniques.

Some dreadlock artists also create custom-made extensions, while others will direct you to their favorite creators and collaborators.

Temporary extensions are an excellent way to get a taste of what it would be like to be a dreadhead without the commitment of a complete installation.

The Beauty of Braid-In Extension

A simple way to "try before you buy in" is to install or have temporary extensions installed in your hair.

This is generally done by sectioning your hair, braiding your natural hair over the extension, and securing it with a rubber band or, in some cases, elastic thread.

Temporary braid-in extensions can be installed over your entire head. You can have them just in the back like you would have partial dreads. Or on a mohawk or at the top of your head if you have shaved sides.

As with natural dreads, your hair needs to be a minimum length for the extensions to be securely in. Three inches is generally a minimum, although many dreadlock artists are willing to install them on shorter hair.

If your hair is long, you don't have to get braid-in extensions the same length as yours. The blanket braid/stitch allows more of your natural hair to be incorporated into the braid, making shorter lengths an option.

Caring for Braid-in Extensions

Temporary braids in extensions are generally not meant to be kept in one's hair for more than 12 weeks/3 months. After that, you'll want to take them out and reinstall them.

You would wash your hair with extensions similar to how you would wash your hair with natural dreads, 1 - 2 times a week, focusing on your scalp.

When you take your extensions out, It is a good idea to wash them gently to remove any debris that may not have washed out when they were in your head.

You can carefully trim off any frizz and generally refresh them before putting them back in or putting them away to use later.

Well-kept extensions can be used and reused multiple times before needing to be retired.

Chapter Eight

WHEN THINGS GO WRONG

I wish that I could tell you that having dreadlocks is all sunshine and rainbows. Sometimes it is. But more often, there are hiccups along the way.

The good news is that there is usually a solution for most problems you encounter as you go along your dreading journey.

Dissatisfaction with Your Locks

How to deal with this will totally depend on when this occurs in your locking journey. If it is early on, as I mentioned above, it may be natural "buyer's remorse." This is especially true if you had your locks done by a professional dreadlock artist whose work you admire. It will pass.

If that isn't the case, try to figure out what is bothering you about your locks. Is it:

- The sizing

- The parting

- The way that the dreads look/feel

- The length

The way the dreads look and feel might be able to be fixed with crocheting. Length can be added. If they are too small, they may be able to be combined without needing to start over.

If you hate the parts or feel they are too thick/big. You may need to remove them and start over again. But don't worry, it can be done, and if your dreads are less than a year old, it should be pretty straightforward. More on dreadlock removal is below.

Thinning/Weak Dreads

What to do about thinning dreads will depend on where they are thinning. At the roots, it could be over-maintenance, hormonal changes (pregnancy, medication, age-related), or heavy extensions.

Improper maintenance methods/sessions, wearing tight beads, bands, or wraps can cause thinning along the length of your dreads.

Once you determine what is causing the problem, it is easier to know how to fix it. If possible, stop or correct what caused it. The actual thin or weak spots along the dreads can be corrected with crochet maintenance.

Mold in Your Dreads

This is one of those issues where prevention is better than cure. You want to avoid having your dreads damp for extended periods.

Once the mold is in your dreads, evidenced by having locks that have a dank, musty odor similar to that of a wet towel. Then the job is to kill the mold.

Due to the nature of dreadlocks, even after the mold is dead, it is hard, if not impossible, to totally remove it from the inside of your lock.

Super Skinny Dreads

If you feel your dreads are too small, you don't necessarily need to start over. It is possible to combine locks using crochet repair techniques. When done correctly, you will be unable to distinguish combined dreads from natural dreads of the same size.

Again prevention is better than cure. To avoid dreads that are too small for your hair or lifestyle, check out the section on sectioning above.

Loopy Bumpy Dreads

This isn't always a bad thing. Some people like dreads that have a little bit more "character." But if your loops and bumps steal the show, they can generally be fixed with crochet maintenance. The age of your dreads will determine how much you'll totally remove them.

Propper tangling at the beginning will significantly reduce the occurrence of loops and bumps as the dreads mature.

Lumps and bumps can be removed with a bit of patience, lock stretching, and palm rolling when wet. This can also help with dreads that have flattened.

Frizzy Locks

This is kinda par for the course. The frizz will go away, at least that frizz along the body of the dread, as your locks mature. Palm rolling after washing can help, especially when your locks are new.

Avoid the temptation of putting tons of products on your dreads in an attempt to "keep the frizz down." What goes on needs to come off sometime. And you will actually start a vicious cycle of scrubbing your dreads to remove the product that will make them frizz more and then putting more product to keep down the frizz.

Products lead to build-up, which can contribute to mold. Not good.

And DO NOT trim the frizz with scissors. Doing so can affect the integrity of your dreads over time as you accidentally cut the hairs that form the mesh that make up your dreads. Just resist the temptation.

All locks are a bit frizzy at times. It's ok. It is just a part of being a dreadhead.

Uneven Dreads

If you have dreads of different lengths and want them more consistent, dreadlock extensions are a good option.

Or, if you are ready for a change, you can always have your dreads cut to make them more even.

Removing Dreadlocks

Yes, dreadlocks can be removed without cutting off all of your hair. I've done it with my own sets, once on 60+ almost 3-year-old locks and again on 350+ 6-month-old locks.

It isn't quick or easy, but it can be done. It will usually take 2 - 3 times longer to take them out than put them in, especially if they are mature.

The oldest areas, those closest to the ends, will be the most challenging to remove. You may want to consider trimming/cutting a few inches off to make the take-down easier if your locks are mature and long.

Some people's hair reacts better to being unraveled dry, while others need heavy use of conditioner to get the dreads out. ONE METHOD DOESN'T FIT ALL. It is worth doing some test dread removal before dumping the bottle of conditioner on your head.

Sometimes oils work better than a conditioner or go completely dry.

A helpful tool to help with removal can be found in the craft section with the loom knitting supplies. It is a loom knitting tool. It works like the end of a rat tail comb, but it is easier to hold and use.

Chapter Nine

How We Help People Get Beautiful Dreads

I hope by now you can see how starting your dreads on the right foundations and proper ongoing maintenance can lead you to have a beautiful head of dreads.

Choosing the right partner to help you start or maintain your dreads can be challenging. Professional dreadlock artists or locticians specializing in straight and wavy hair are few and far between. It is tempting to throw your hands up and let anyone do your hair or do your best to DIY when you'd rather not.

It is worth seeking out a professional dreadlock artist. Doing so can help you start your dreadlocking journey better or get you on the right track if your dreads started out less than ideal.

We Give Educated Guidance

Most professional dreadlock artists have completed specialized training to hone their skills in this craft. Some have apprenticed with other master locticians. Others have taken on and offline courses. Others have brought their background in formal hair education to their work with dreads.

For many of us, this is the focus of our business. So we are invested in being our best and providing the guidance and education to help our clients have the best dreading experience possible.

We Share Informed Suggestions

It is one thing to google, "what to do when _____." It is another thing to have a professional look at your dreads, understand your background, goals, and lifestyle, and give suggestions specific to your situation.

There are few one-size-fits-all answers. And what may work for someone else whose hair may resemble yours may not work best for you.

Everyone is different. We consider those differences when seeking to provide you with an experience tailored for you and your hair.

We Provide Empathetic Support

Most dreadlock artists have or have had dreadlocks of some type at some point in their lives. Our own dreadlocking journeys may have been the spark for our decision to provide the service to others.

So we can empathize with you. We get it because we've been through it and helped others.

Chapter Ten

The Next Step

Congratulations! You are one step closer to dreadfully beautiful hair. I hope I have opened your eyes to the possibilities of starting and maintaining locs with straight or wavy hair. And hopefully, you are excited about the potential of working with me or another professional dreadlock artist.

Think about your satisfaction when someone tells you, "I love your dreads! They are so beautiful!"

Feel the joy of waking up and going without needing to give a second thought to what you need to do to your hair.

Trust me, it is gratifying and will make you wonder why you didn't make the decision to loc your hair sooner.

Don't Lose Your Momentum

As I mentioned earlier in the book, I wrote it for two primary reasons:

1. To help, inspire and motivate readers like you;

2. To extend an invitation to see if getting professional help with dreading your hair makes sense for all parties involved.

Let me ask you to consider these three questions and answer them in your mind.

1. Would having locs installed bring you closer to the vision of yourself that you see in your mind?

2. Are you ready to commit to having your hair dreaded installed and up for the changes that may come with your hair and life?

3. Do you value working with an expert to start your locking journey, guide you along the path to bring out the best in your hair, and help you prevent mishaps and mistakes?

If your answers are three yeses, then you really have three pathways in front of you at this very moment.

1. You can close this book and do nothing with the information I shared. (If you have gotten this far, I sure hope this isn't an option ;-))

2. You can start your dreads on your own by leveraging the tips, tactics, and strategies I have just given you.

3. By reaching out to a professional dreadlock artist, you can ensure that your dreads are started off on a solid foundation.

If you are serious about having dreads that look good and that last, you have nothing to lose by choosing the third pathway.

Once you've decided, you are open to exploring the possibility of getting professional help. The next step would be to reach out and book a consultation.

You'll usually be asked to fill out a form before speaking with someone. This allows us to understand what is going on with your dreads. It lets us see what you hope to achieve with a new installation.

It is always good to be as thorough as possible when filling out the consultation form.

You'll usually be asked to submit photos of your dreads from various angles and possibly inspirational images of what you hope your dreads will look like.

Depending on the artist, after the form is filled out, you may be sent to a page to book a time, or they may reach out to you when they have time.

Bibliography

Bailey, Diane Carol. *Milady Standard Natural Hair Care & Braiding*. Milady, a Part of Cengage Learning, 2014.

Bansen, Erika. "FAQ." *Make Me Dreadful*, http://www.makemedreadful.biz/faq.

Bilal-Ali, Aishah. "Loctician Certification Online School." *Natural Hair Class*, https://www.naturalhairclass.com/bundles/loctician-certification.

Bonner, Lonnie Brittenum. *Nice Dreads: Hair Care Basics and Inspiration for Colored Girls Who've Considered Locking Their Hair*. Three Rivers Press, 2005.

Colby. "Dreadlock FAQ: All Your Dreadlock Questions Finally Answered." *Dreadlock Central*, 6 June 2020, https://dreadlockcentral.com/faq-dreadlock-questions/.

"Dreadlock Education ." *Alternative Hairstyles, Dreadlocks & Maintenance*, Avani Joy, 2013, https://www.ragingrootsstudio.com/dreadlock-education/.

"Dreadlock FAQ." *Rebel Rebel Philly Hair and Dreadlock Salon*, https://www.rebelrebelphilly.com/dreadlocks-faq.

"Dreadlock FAQ." *Southern Dreadlocks*, https://www.southerndreadlocks.com.au/faq.

Evans, Nekena. *Hairlocking: Everything You Need to Know African, Dread & Nubian Locks*. Eworld Inc, 2010.

Fleming, JoAnna. *LIFE LESSONS & LOCS: Loose Natural Hair Confessions & Loc Maintenance Lessons*. JoAnna Fleming, 2020.

George, M. Michele. *The Knotty Truth: Creating Beautiful Locks on a Dime!: A Comprehensive Guide to Creating Locks*. Manifest Publishing Enterprises, 2010.

Illingworth, Kimberly Ann. *Dreadlocks: The Sacred Hair*. Independently Published, 2020.

Jacob Cohen. "Dreadlocks Denver FAQ." *Dreadlocks Denver*, 22 Apr. 2022, https://www.dreadlocksdenver.com/dreadlocks-denver-faq/.

"Kris McDred Loctician." *Kris McDred*, 26 Apr. 2022, https://krismcdred.com/kris-mcdred-loctician/.

Liong-A-Kong, Mireille. *Going Natural How to Fall in Love with Nappy Hair*. Sabi Wiri, 2004.

Liz Kidder Studio. "Dreadlocks. Accessories. Education." *Liz Kidder Studio*, https://lizkidderstudio.com/.

Making Dreadlocks Using a Tool. Nappylocs, 2015.

Marjolein. "Saltydreads." *SaltyDreads*, http://www.saltydreads.com/.

Mastalia, Francesco, and Alfonse Pagano. *Dreads*. Artisan, 2000.

Willemse, Xima. *FAQ*, https://www.dreadxshop.com/faq.

Acknowledgments

This book wouldn't be possible if it were not for many people's support, encouragement, and inspiration.

To my husband, Conrad McKnight, my daughter Amelia McKnight, my mom Rose Knight and my brother Phil Knight when I have a project, I'm like a dog with a bone. Thank you for checking in, helping out, listening, and being patient with me as I finished this.

To Ms. Latonya Evans, owner/director of the Millinemum Trade Academy, thanks for working with my schedule so that I could complete the program and get legal ;-). And all the MTA staff: Ms. Marion, Ms. Jones,

CJ, and Aunt Bert. Thanks for the encouragement and support that helped me pass my written and practical exams on the first try. To my amazing classmates, Kenielle, Ayanna, Ebony, and Monica, I learned from each of you.

To the fantastic straight and wavy-haired ladies who trusted me to do their dreads and braids: Kristy Marshall, Erin Hardy, Stacy Yokely, Cynthia Hall, Amanda Abarca, and Kaitlyn Frye, you all are the reason I wrote this book!

To my locking mentor, Kris McDred, thank you for putting out that first youtube video. I was one of the millions that watched it many years ago and used it to instant loc, my first client. Who knew I'd get to learn directly from the source? Thank you for encouraging us all to master locking.

To Rob Fitzpatrick, Adam Rosen, and the Monday and Wednesday Writing Accountability Group members. You pushed me to outdo what I did last, lol. I may have quit if I didn't know you all might miss my reports ;-)

DREADFUL BEAUTY

To Mike Capuzzi, your books and podcast were my guides along the way. I am looking forward to working with you on a future book.

To Matt Rudnitsky, your book allowed me to stop making excuses and finish the thing!

Finally, to all my new friends, beta readers, and podcast guest on Instagram:

Avani Visone (agingrootsstudio), Rebecca Cengiz-Robbs (rebaweaves), Libby (blissfulzeal), Jennifer Leigh Sørum (earthymamawitch), Nomadic Dreads NZ (nomadic_dreads), Lauren (Locs_of_Loz), Heather Nealson (dalydreads), Bert (therrukest), Wanderlust Dreadlocks (wanderlust_locs), Aubrey Mccollum (aubrey_velvetlockslounge), Kayla Lussier (limelightstudiollc), Kathleen Anne Tamburrano (red_forrest_dreads), Zara (zara_locksfromlove), Britt Peat (hippieishginger), Tanis Clay (tanis.gem.tone), Sarah Burks (greenthumblady), and Angie Gomez (MorbidLocs)

Thanks for reading the first drafts, giving feedback, sharing your stories on the podcast, and generally welcoming me into a world that is very different from the locking world I had previously known.

If I missed anyone, count it to my head and not my heart, and let me know so I can update the next edition!

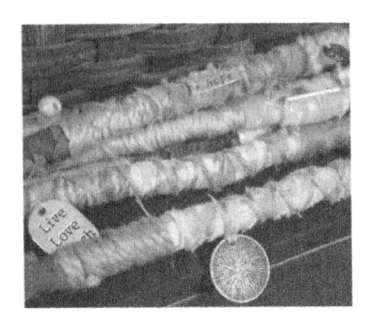

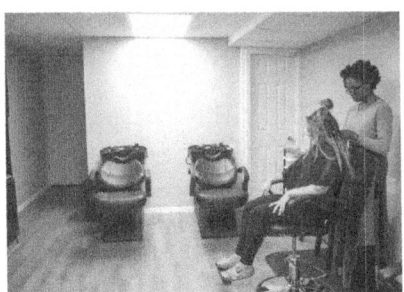

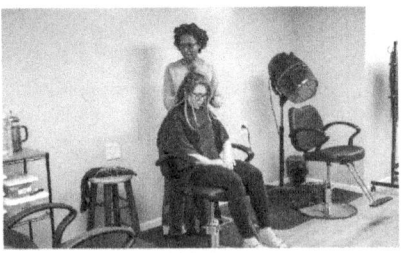

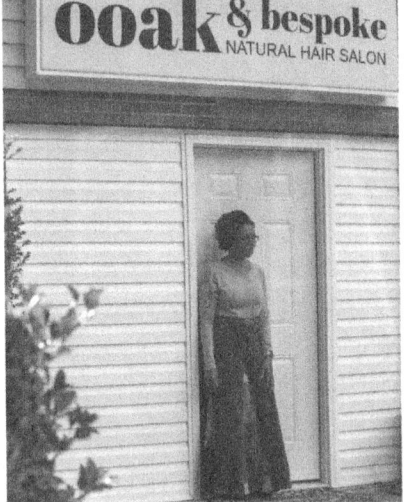

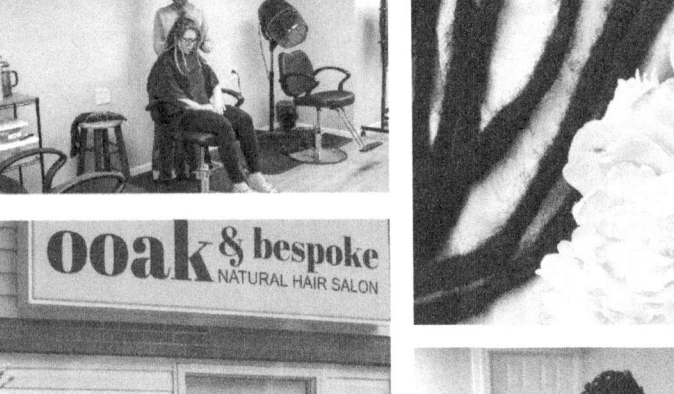

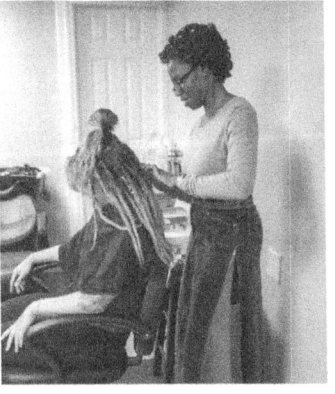

Model: Kristy Marshal
Photographer: Erin Hardy, Hardy Photography

About Amy McKnight

Amy McKnight is a Licensed Natural Hair Care Specialist and Dreadlock Artist living in Lexington, North Carolina. She specializes in product-free dreadlock installation and maintenance using various methods based on her client's lifestyles, hair types, and ultimate goals for having locks.

She has had natural locks or worn some type of faux dreadlock style on and off for over 20 years. She was an editor and principal contributor for MyNHCG.com, formally NaturalHairCareGuide.com, where she wrote dozens of articles on dreadlocks and hair locking.

Amy has done hair on and off as a side business for over a decade. When she learned that licensing is required in North Carolina, where she resides, she returned to school to get the required certification. She then opened a state-licensed 2-chair salon, OOAK & Bespoke, in her home.

Before making the career switch to entirely focus on dread care, she taught creative rigid heddle weaving on and offline. She enjoys fiber arts and yarn crafting and loves being able to bring that background into what she does with her clients.

She and her husband Conrad own a successful computer repair and sales business. Where she worked for ten years before switching to hair. They have one daughter, one dog, one guinea pig, 4 gerbils, and 3 freshwater fish.

For more information on working with Amy, you can reach out to her via her website: www.ooakandbespok.com. You'll find a list of the services she offers and book a consultation call to speak with her about possibly starting your dreads.

Also By Amy McKnight

Freedom in Locs

Interlock Love (Coming 2023)

Tendrilocs: Next Generation Micro-Sized Braid Locs (Coming 2023)

About the Dreadful Beauty Podcast

The Dreadful Beauty Podcast is an interview-style podcast with host Amy McKnight, dreadlock artists, women who wear dreadlocks, and businesses who support them.

Each episode shares information, encouragement, and support for women who wear, want, or love dreadlocks. If you are looking for a virtual community to encourage you or like to learn more about a potential partner in your journey, tune into the show!

Listen on Spotify. Just type in "Dreadful Beauty"

A Small Request

Thank you so much for reading *Dreadful Beauty*! If you follow this book's information, I'm positive that you will have amazingly beautiful dreads.

When you do, please send me a selfie. I'd love to see how your dreads came out! My email is on the next page ;-)

I have a small, quick favor to ask. Would you mind taking a minute or two and sending me an honest review of this book? Reviews are the BEST way to help others find out about this book, and I read all my reviews looking for helpful feedback. Visit:

OOAKandBespoke.com/books

Click the book's name, and you'll see a link to leave a review! Thank you in advance!

Made in the USA
Columbia, SC
08 October 2022